first place
4health

2009
journal

Published by Gospel Light
Ventura, California, U.S.A.
www.gospellight.com
Printed in the U.S.A.

Rights for publishing this book outside the U.S.A. or in non-English languages are administered by Gospel Light Worldwide, an international not-for-profit ministry. For additional information, please visit www.glww.org, email info@glww.org, or write to Gospel Light Worldwide, 1957 Eastman Avenue, Ventura, CA 93003, U.S.A.

the importance of journaling

I began writing in a prayer journal in 1990, and this habit has dramatically impacted my life. In the beginning, I wrote three to four pages a day, because God was teaching me to be consistent in prayer. On those pages, I shared what was going on in my life and asked God to help me that day to do His will.

I used my prayer journal in this way until 1997, when we moved from Houston to Galveston Bay. This move dramatically changed the way that I use my journal. Before, when I had lived only three miles from the First Place office, I had plenty of time to write. Now I lived 46 miles from work, and I had to get up an hour earlier than I had before the move. I was so frustrated at not having the time to write, and during the next couple of years, I floundered in my prayer life because I wanted things to be the same as they had been when I first began writing my prayers. In a sense, I had made a god out of writing in my journal.

One day, a friend taught me a new way to pray. Jeannie Blocher, founder of Body & Soul Aerobics, and I were in Ventura, California, for a meeting with our publisher. Body & Soul was going to produce the first exercise DVD for our program, and we had some very important meetings scheduled that day. Jeannie and I went out for a walk, and Jeannie said, "Why don't we pray as we walk?" I had prayed on the phone with people, and I had prayed corporately in church, but this was absolutely the first time I had ever done this type of prayer. Jeannie prayed for a while, and then I began praying. We continued this way until we finished our walk an hour later.

God showed me an important principle that morning: It doesn't matter how you pray; you simply must do it. So today, I use my journal in a completely different way. I write about the big problems going on in my life. I write about situations at work in which I need God's wisdom. I write about the specific ways that God answers my prayers. I pray aloud during the 46-mile drive into Houston each morning, and I do my writing on the weekends when I have more time. I write about funny stories that I might want to use later when I write a book. The idea is that for one year, my life is between the pages of my journal.

My journal is just as important today as it was all those years ago when I first began writing my prayers, even though the form and method has changed. My prayer for you is that you will enjoy your journal and make it your friend during this coming year. You might like to use it for writing your prayers, or you might like to divide it into four sections and write about how God is helping you find balance mentally, spiritually, emotionally and physically. I like to make a list in the back of my journal of people who have asked me to pray for them. I don't list all of my family members, because I remember their names, but it is easy to forget about people if I don't write their names down.

I hope you enjoy your journal this year. I know I will enjoy mine.

Carole Lewis
First Place 4 Health National Director

The river of the Spirit of God overcomes all obstacles.
Never get your eyes on the obstacle or on the difficulty.

OSWALD CHAMBERS

Do not have your concert first, and then tune your instrument afterwards. Begin the day with the Word of God and prayer, and get first of all into harmony with Him.

HUDSON TAYLOR

By perseverance the snail reached the ark.
CHARLES SPURGEON

One life yielded to God at all costs is worth thousands only touched by God.

Oswald Chambers

In all ranks of life the human heart yearns for the beautiful; and the beautiful things that God makes are his gift to all alike.

HARRIET BEECHER STOWE

You are never too old to set another goal or to dream a new dream.
C.S. LEWIS

_____

_____

_____

_____

_____

_____

_____

_____

_____

_____

_____

_____

_____

_____

_____

_____

_____

_____

_____

_____

It is not the passing of the years that matures the life of the Son of God in us, but obedience.

OSWALD CHAMBERS

_____

_____

_____

_____

_____

_____

_____

_____

_____

_____

_____

_____

_____

_____

_____

_____

_____

_____

_____

_____

_____

He that lives in hope dances without music.
GEORGE HERBERT

You pay God a compliment by asking great things of Him.

TERESA OF ÁVILA

If once we accept the revelation of Jesus Christ that God is our Father and that we can never think of anything He will forget, worry becomes impossible.

OSWALD CHAMBERS

God, who touchest earth with beauty, make me lovely too;
with Thy Spirit re-create me, make my heart anew.

MARY S. EDGAR

_____

_____

_____

_____

_____

_____

_____

_____

_____

_____

_____

_____

_____

_____

_____

_____

_____

_____

_____

Prayer—secret, fervent, believing prayer—
lies at the root of all personal godliness.
WILLIAM CAREY

Character is always revealed in crisis.

OSWALD CHAMBERS

Not for one single day, can I discern my way, but this
I surely know—Who gives the day will show the way.

JOHN OXENHAM

Cheerfulness, it would appear, is a matter which depends fully as much on the state of things within, as on the state of things without and around us.

CHARLOTTE BRONTË

"Present your bodies . . ." Do not ask God to take
your body, but give your body to God.
OSWALD CHAMBERS

He became what we are that He might make us what He is.

ATHANASIUS

_____

_____

_____

_____

_____

_____

_____

_____

_____

_____

_____

_____

_____

_____

_____

_____

_____

_____

_____

In this world of tribulation . . . He will keep you in perfect peace . . .
Whose mind is stayed on [Him].
RICHARD J. OLIVER

God never allows a Christian to carry on his life in sections . . .
the whole life, spirit, soul and body must progress together.

OSWALD CHAMBERS

_____

_____

_____

_____

_____

_____

_____

_____

_____

_____

_____

_____

_____

_____

_____

_____

_____

_____

_____

God, give me sympathy and sense, and help me keep my courage high;
God, give me calm and confidence, and—please—a twinkle in my eye.

MARGARET BAILEY

_____

_____

_____

_____

_____

_____

_____

_____

_____

_____

_____

_____

_____

_____

_____

_____

_____

Jesus Christ is the Completer of unfinished people.
LONA M. FOWLER

_____

_____

_____

_____

_____

_____

_____

_____

_____

_____

_____

_____

_____

_____

_____

_____

_____

_____

_____

_____

_____

_____

It is a life of FAITH, not of intellect and reason,
but a life of knowing Who makes us.
OSWALD CHAMBERS

I walk in wonders beyond myself.
C. S. LEWIS

One can never consent to creep when one feels an impulse to soar.

HELEN KELLER

Forgiveness is the divine miracle of grace.

OSWALD CHAMBERS

Never give up, for that is just the place and time that the tide will turn.
HARRIET BEECHER STOWE

When we have exhausted our store of endurance, when our strength has failed ere the day is half done . . . Our Father's full giving is only begun.

ANNIE JOHNSON FLINT

_____

_____

_____

_____

_____

_____

_____

_____

_____

_____

_____

_____

_____

_____

_____

_____

_____

_____

_____

Remember, we go through nothing that God does not know about.
OSWALD CHAMBERS

_____

_____

_____

_____

_____

_____

_____

_____

_____

_____

_____

_____

_____

_____

_____

_____

_____

_____

_____

_____

Through every minute of this day, be with me, Lord!
JOHN OXENHAM

Attitude determines altitude.

ANONYMOUS

*It is not what a man achieves, but what he believes
and strives for that makes him noble and great.*

OSWALD CHAMBERS